AUTHORITY IN MEDICINE:
OLD AND NEW

AUTHORITY IN MEDICINE:
OLD AND NEW

BY

MAJOR GREENWOOD

D.Sc., F.R.C.P., F.R.S.

Professor of Epidemiology and Vital Statistics
in the University of London

THE LINACRE LECTURE

6 MAY 1943

CAMBRIDGE

AT THE UNIVERSITY PRESS

1943

CAMBRIDGE
UNIVERSITY PRESS

University Printing House, Cambridge CB2 8BS, United Kingdom

Published in the United States of America by Cambridge University Press, New York

Cambridge University Press is part of the University of Cambridge.

It furthers the University's mission by disseminating knowledge in the pursuit of education, learning and research at the highest international levels of excellence.

www.cambridge.org
Information on this title: www.cambridge.org/9781107664982

© Cambridge University Press 1943

First published 1943
Re-issued 2014

A catalogue record for this publication is available from the British Library

ISBN 978-1-107-66498-2 Paperback

AUTHORITY IN MEDICINE:
OLD AND NEW

AN INVITATION from the Master and Fellows of St John's College to prepare this lecture brought me satisfaction of a kind which a majority of the audience cannot experience. I have known and loved Cambridge in general and St John's College in particular for many years, but my memories are largely of vacations. You will recall Charles Lamb on Oxford in vacation: 'Here I can take my walks unmolested, and fancy myself of what degree or standing I please. I seem admitted ad eundem. I fetch up past opportunities. I can rise at the chapel-bell and dream that it rings for *me*. In moods of humility I can be a Sizar or Servitor. When the peacock vein rises, I strut a Gentleman Commoner. In graver moments, I proceed Master of Arts.' My memories are not quite those of Elia, for I have known Cambridge in term and even had a tiny share in her teaching; but more akin to his than to those of her sons and daughters. My memories are of week-ends and haunt a set of rooms in the Second Court of St John's where, thirty years ago, a young week-end visitor eagerly listened to his host's account of Cambridge life and, if he did not actually break the 10th Commandment, was certainly more conscious of the advantages than of the drawbacks of Collegiate life.

The, no longer, young week-end visitor takes pleasure in the thought that his name has secured that degree of permanent association with St John's College which entry on the College roll of memorial lecturers confers. Some lecturer may idly wonder whom this forgotten name denoted and what the predecessor had written, but will hardly satisfy so faint a curiosity. Few lecturers are like the profound classical scholar who, Sir Thomas Watson tells us, 'was possessed with the strange curiosity to read all the printed Harveian Orations' and found very few 'the latinity of which he could praise'.

That Sir Thomas Watson—once a Linacre Lecturer—characterises this zeal as a 'strange curiosity' is not encouraging; a President of the College of Physicians, he had heard a great many Harveian Orations. I have not equalled the industry of the profound classical scholar, but have read a good many Harveian Orations. The variates of my sample had this common feature. *All* the lecturers expressed a high opinion of Harvey; many of them devoted much of their space to a study of some aspect of Harvey's work or of its bearing upon the progress of medical science. My sampling of printed Linacre Lectures has been smaller and the resulting inferences subject to a large error of sampling. But, in my small sample, the merits of the pious founder are not always emphasised.

In 1922 Sir Humphry Rolleston politely observed that, as Sir William Osler had sympathetically considered Linacre in 1908, he need do no more than attempt the briefest reference. In 1928 Sir George Newman did gracefully praise Linacre, but the tribute paid in 1940 to the pious memory of the founder by my old friend and former colleague Dr Topley* reminded me of the lines:

'A while like one in dreams he stood,
Then faltered forth his gratitude
In words just short of being rude.'

Topley spoke kindly of Linacre as a scholar but: 'As a physician, I cannot avoid the conclusion that the only reason he did no more harm than he did was because the times were too much for him.' Linacre 'spent his labour in putting a brighter polish on the fetters that held medicine in thrall'.

Topley's opinion was that Linacre believed the science of medicine to have been perfected by the Greek physicians and that Galen's works crystallised their conclusive wisdom, so that the primary need of his time was to diffuse accurate knowledge of the ancient treatises.

It *is* certain that Linacre attached great importance to the preparation of a correct and readable translation of Galen's works and himself made valuable contributions to this task. But little else is certain. Our knowledge of Linacre is shadowy. We have a portrait of him and a fairly precise record of his academic career and of his numerous preferments. We have appraisements of his intellectual and ethical qualities by good judges who knew and admired him, even by one, a professor in this university, Cheke, who did *not* greatly admire him. But Linacre

* W. W. C. Topley, *Authority, Observation and Experiment in Medicine*, Cambridge (U.P.), 1940.

as a human being is hidden from us. Of his personal correspondence one, quite uninformative, letter[1] remains. We do know that he was human enough to quarrel with a friend who thought a book he had written too hard for schoolboys, but what he really thought of the future of medicine, what were his dreams and aspirations, is matter for guess-work. My guess has no more intrinsic value than Topley's, but is different.

However great our admiration of the heuristic method, even now we admit the use of text-books. If respect for authority means accepting the assertions of a teacher whom we believe (without being good judges) to be competent, even now the most independent-minded of medical students bow to authority. The medical curriculum is lengthy; it would be still longer if, for instance, every student verified experimentally text-book statements on the properties and dosages of all the relatively few drugs which are still esteemed. What we try to do is to encourage students to verify experimentally some statements and to put into their hands only text-books all the statements of which have been verified by competent persons.

Linacre must have found that the text-books of his student days were bad, but that they purported to record the opinions and reasonings of Galen. There was a Galenical faith, just as there is now a Marxian faith, and medical students at the end of the fifteenth century were no more familiar with the words of Galen than young English sectaries of Marx with *his* opinions; they were probably less familiar with them, Galen wrote much more than Marx and had been far less accurately translated. Linacre was familiar with Galen's writings. The problem he had to solve as an educational reformer was whether Galen's teachings were so bad that no selection of his writings could be made into an elementary text-book, that a root and branch reform was imperative, or whether Galen not as a vague oracle but as a writer known at least at second-hand might be a useful teacher. If Linacre as an educational reformer, like Burke as a political reformer, shrank from violent changes his bias would be towards a use of Galen. The question is whether Linacre's conclusion was wrong. This involves a consideration of what kind of writer Galen was.

Nobody who reads Galen now is in danger of the bias with which the idol of a powerful class must be judged; the enemy of mankind has, however, set two traps for him. These, as usual with Satan's most effective methods, are baited to catch vanity; herd vanity and personal vanity. If one discovers that an ancient writer had reached some conclusion similar to our own on a matter which still interests us, herd vanity assures one that he must have been a very superior man. Individual vanity prompts us to make rather too much of the (to us) hitherto unknown merits of a writer we have read with difficulty; it is not pleasant to think that we have been wasting our time, that the ignorant world is wiser than we. I suppose I show the teeth marks of both traps. During the last twenty-five years, at odd moments, I have read a fair amount of

Galen's work (2), say 15 per cent of it carefully and another 10 per cent cursorily, including two of the three larger treatises Linacre translated. I avoided Galen's anatomical works and concentrated on his epidemiology, general hygiene and medical psychology.

The first thing which occurs to a modern reader is that Galen was almost comically unlike one's idea of an oracle or a prophet. He had certainly two characteristics in common with the Hebrew prophets, viz. an extremely low opinion of most of his contemporaries and an immense command of the vocabulary of vituperation; also, at times, a beauty of phrasing which still glows faintly in translation. Thus he reproved a writer who, he said, ignored the creative power of Nature and adds: 'Aristotle, dealing with this very subject, wondered whether there were not a beginning more divine, something other than just heat and cold and moist and dry. Wherefore I think it wrong of men to draw such rash conclusions in matters so great and to assign to the qualities alone the power of shaping the parts. It may be these are nothing more than instruments and something else the master hand' (*de Temperamentis*, Bk. 2, Kühn, vol. 1, pp. 635–6). There the resemblance ends. Galen was emphatically not the prophet of the Most High God, dictating commandments; he was for ever giving reasons, he was sometimes witty, often abusive, but always arguing. If he conceived himself to be a dictator (there is no reason to think he did) he was guilty of the imprudence Bagehot attributed to John Milton, who made God argue, with the inevitable consequence that later generations would dis-cover God did not argue very well.

Galen's epidemiological influence was, I think, bad be-cause he over-rated the creative power not of Nature but of his own intelligence. He skilfully developed a formal description of epidemic phenomena, a description which actually did describe the phenomena and explain why epidemics rose, declined and fell, so neatly that men might easily think the problem solved (3). He never con-sidered alternative hypotheses and deserves blame for that because the demography and medical statistics of Imperial Rome were at least as well documented as those of London in the sixteenth and seventeenth centuries. Had Galen been less proud of his intellect, he could have done as much as John Graunt, a humble-minded researcher, did 1500 years later. We can hardly blame Galen's mediaeval pupils, who had no demographic data of value, for not doing what he left undone.

Galen's treatise on personal hygiene, one of the longer works translated by Linacre, is probably the most readable and illuminating of his books. It is not tediously long—a modern translation would run perhaps to 250 octavo pages—and could easily be reduced in bulk by omitting repetitions; Galen's sense of literary form was not Platonic. The proportion of repulsively obsolete technicality is small. Within the limits he defines, Galen's advice would be regarded by most physicians as excellent. The narrow-ness of the limits, however, shocks our humanity. Early in his treatise, Galen tells the reader that a great majority of mankind live 'encumbered by affairs which must need injure those engaged in them, and cannot change their condition'. Some are poor, some slaves, some unintelligent. 'To lay down rules of hygiene for such persons is idle. But if anyone by luck or design is free, to him it is proper to describe how he may be healthy, may be tried as little as possible by disease and may grow old agreeably' (Kühn, VI, 82).

Having thus limited the discussion to a small minority, viz. to persons who can command the services not only of physicians but gymnastic instructors, architects, cooks and personal servants, he gives an admirable exposition of practical dietetics, physical training and the Horatian philosophy of life. The importance of moderation, the need to distrust general formulae, to study the individual are emphasised in a way which would surprise a reader who has supposed Galen to be a dogmatist—in the modern sense of the word *not* the Galenical sense. A modern reader may object that while Galen's practical advice is sound, his reasons for the advice are nonsensical. For instance, while his remark that to give a boy wine can do him no good and must do him harm is morally and medically sound (Kühn, VI, 55), the explanation, that the humoural type of children is humid and this deviation is exacerbated by alcohol, is nonsense. But—quite apart from the danger of misinterpretation which a changing connotation of technical words brings—one feels that these 'reasons' are often either rationalisations in the modern sense, or simply a framework of reference, a kind of mnemonic which helps Galen, and perhaps his readers, to retain in an orderly way knowledge which has been gained by experience. He makes the significant remark: 'I always teach that in the art of medicine, reasoning may easily find an explanation; belief comes from experience' (Kühn, VI, 368).

If Linacre thought this treatise a sound introduction to the study of personal hygiene, I see no reason to dissent from his opinion.

As a medical psychologist, Galen was in advance of any medical writers of the Renaissance age (4).

His chief psychological work, *de Placitis*, the only one of his major writings available in a modern critical edition (Mueller's) (5), probably never had many medical readers. It is very long and to a modern reader the Stoic doctrine that πάθη, Cicero's *perturbationes*, St Thomas Aquinas' *passiones animae*, our *affects*, have their origin wholly in faulty intellectual processes and can be corrected by wholly intellectual, cognitive methods, does not now seem to need refutation. Indeed, one is apt to suspect that the Stoic theory could not have been so silly as Galen seems to say it was. Reference, however, to the *Tusculan Disputations*—the work of a disciple not a critic of Stoicism—does not confirm the suspicion. 'Totus vero iste qui vulgo appellatur amor—nec invenio quo nomine alio possit appellari—tantae levitatis est, ut nihil videam quod putem conferendum' is a fine phrase, but an odd one in the mouth of a man whose career was destroyed by affects *his* excellent intellect could never control. Galen did realise that the clinical treatment of psychoneuroses needed sympathetic insight and, had his 'authority' prevailed, the volume of psychoneurotic misery might have been diminished a few centuries sooner. That all he knew and all St Thomas Aquinas knew—a good deal more than Galen—has been independently re-discovered, does not alter the fact that Galen was a much better medical psychologist than most medical successors down to very modern times.

If I have *fairly* characterised the work of Galen, then, in my view, Linacre in retaining some of Galen's writings as text-books did not convict himself of authoritarianism in the disparaging sense of the word, viz. as used by Topley. But a closer examination of what we do mean by authority in science is needed.

The emotional attitude which compels one to believe that what A said is true and to decline even to examine evidence that what A said is false can have no defenders among men of science. But I doubt whether it *ever* greatly influenced men inquisitive enough and intelligent enough to discover any new truth. Such men as Galen and Thomas Aquinas, who professed enormous reverence for authority—Galen for that of Hippocrates, Thomas for that of Aristotle—will often be found attributing to their professed masters their own, original opinions.

Most modern authors speak with a special contempt of the Scholastics. Linacre's biographer, Johnson, is eloquent on that theme. My casual reading of these derided thinkers leads to me conclude that they were neither less intelligent nor more subservient to authority than the anatomists and physiologists of the Renaissance, but only that they were interested in a different way of satisfying their intellectual curiosity.

With us a special prestige attaches to the experimental method. We all feel that an experimental 'proof' or test has more authority to bind than any other intellectual procedure. One's heart warms at the thought of a *crucial* experiment. Thirty-eight years ago as a junior demonstrator of physiology I assisted my professor in researches into the effects of high barometric pressure on animals. It had been proved years earlier by Paul Bert that the efficient cause of Caisson Disease and Divers' Palsy was the liberation of nitrogen bubbles from solution in the tissues; the object of my professor's researches was to improve methods of decompression in industrial work. It occurred to me that if one exposed to high pressure simultaneously an animal with and an animal without a blood respiratory system, and decompressed them suddenly, the former would die and the latter survive. I immured a frog, a goat moth caterpillar and a cork in a glass chamber, raised the pressure, watched my prisoners for ten minutes or so, then decompressed them suddenly and experienced an Archimedean thrill when the frog went into convulsions and died while the caterpillar still crawled care-free over the cork (it subsequently pupated and emerged a normal moth). A crucial experiment indeed. But my professor, had he not been a kindly man, might have said: ' My dear lad, our knowledge of the physiological mechanisms of frogs and caterpillars is extensive. If your experiment does *not* end in the death of the frog and the survival of the caterpillar, the only inference you may draw is that your experiment was inefficiently made.' He would have been right; my experiment added nothing to scientific knowledge, it pleased my vanity and strengthened, *pro tanto*, my emotional faith.

There is perhaps a moral in this trivial incident. We may over-rate the logical value of the experimental method and under-rate its educational or emotional value. *Real* experiments are difficult, unlike the arm-chair experiments of Francis Bacon. A comparison of the rules of *Novum Organum* with Professor R. A. Fisher's *The Design of Experiments* will satisfy most readers that Bacon was not a much more useful teacher, or text-book writer, than the despised ancients. The authority of the experimental method is not intrinsically much more respectable than that of ancient logic. But any biometrician over sixty can remember the contemptuous hostility with which many biological laboratory workers spoke of 'mathematical' methods; the authority of the skilled experimenter was not to be challenged by mathematicians who had never done any experiments at all. That is no longer the attitude of biologists; one finds Raymond Pearl, biologist and bio-metrician, writing: 'Of all methodological procedures in biology, the *experimentum crucis* is the most dangerous. A great deal is heard to the effect that the crucial experiment is the only thing that really counts. All other types of biological methodology are contemptuously characterised as "vague" or worse. But nothing emerges more clearly from the history of biological thought than that, almost without exception, the crucial experiments which have been most loudly hailed at the time they were made, as for ever settling the problem under discussion, have been found to have led to quite erroneous conclusions' (*The Rate of Living*, New York, 1928, pp. 32–3).

Into that field of medical research which has attracted me, epidemiology, Topley introduced the experimental method nearly a quarter of a century ago. For more than fifteen years I had the happiness to be associated with him in the research. Whether my opinion is just, viz. that we discovered some unsuspected factors of epidemic variation, destroyed some fallacious beliefs and verified some hypotheses still not generally accepted, time will decide (6). But the great secrets of epidemiology are still secrets. We still do not know why Scarlet Fever has become almost what Sydenham called it, a mere name of a disease. We still cannot say why Influenza is sometimes a gentle corrective, sometimes an earth-shaking pandemic. Perhaps the scale of our operations was too small. To use the statistical lecturer's stock illustration, we did not draw enough counters from the infinitively large bag; we could not do so for here a counter is not one mouse but one experiment, an experiment involving hundreds of animals and many months of time. We both had an emotional conviction that the danger point in herd-life, the moment when something was likely to happen, depended on an unstable equilibrium, perhaps some critical ratio of num-

17

bers in different categories of herd experience, but we could not clearly define the conditions. Perhaps some reader of our protocols with deeper insight may discern the truth. Perhaps—and self-esteem inclines me to that view—our statistical experience *was* too small. If under a Utopian planning scheme, our methods were applied on a hundred-fold scale, the secrets of epidemic succession in herds of mice might be laid bare. But they would be the secrets of herds of mice; their generalisation to societies of men would remain a task.

Perhaps there is more promise in the plan of campaign of the statistical epidemiologists of the Johns Hopkins School of Public Health, inspired largely by that gifted investigator, the late Wade Hampton Frost (7). They leave the experimental work to Nature, but acquaint themselves thoroughly with the characters of herds in which Nature will make experiments, families of human beings, rich and poor, well housed and ill housed. The precise statistical characterisation of human groups is no new thing. One remembers the work of Booth and Rowntree. It is a question merely of a change of emphasis; the epidemiologists interest themselves primarily in those group characters which might be expected to have a bearing on the rise and fall of epidemic diseases and do not disdain to record 'trifling' ailments. This is slow, tedious work, but, in my submission, it is neither less important nor makes fewer demands on intellectual ability than experimental medicine in the laboratory sense of the term; but its prestige in popular or even scientific circles is far less.

It is possible to over-rate the immediate effect on the public health of laboratory discoveries. When I hear the B.B.C. Announcer say: 'Last night the Royal Air Force carried out a very heavy raid on X' my attention wanders from the following rather vague sentences. I am waiting for the final, definite words: 'N of our machines did not return.' I know there will be more than N fathers and mothers asking:

'Why didst thou leave the trodden path of men
Too soon, and with weak hands though mighty heart
Dare the unpastured dragon in his den?'

And I seek *some* consolation, or distraction. I find it in arithmetic, easily enough, because my own sons are not airmen. I think of the death rates to which young men of 20–25 were subjected when Shelley wrote those words, and for more than a generation longer, and of the death rate in that age group when the war began. I then take the population of young Englishmen, 20–25, as it was in 1939 or 1940 and do this sum: How many young men must die by military violence in this year to bring the quota up to what it would have been had they died at the rates of their great-grandfathers in peaceful times? The answer is 7500; the crews of, say, 1500 bombers a year. Consider two items in the excessive toll of young lives 70 to 100 years ago. Between 1848 and 1873 nearly 190,000 Englishmen aged 20–25 died. Of these, 18,000 died of Typhus and 85,000 of Phthisis. These two items account for more than half the total. Typhus in the civilian population of England and Wales is a pathological curiosity; the mortality from Pulmonary Tuberculosis has been reduced to about one-fifth of what it was.

It is not a mere paradox to say that in 1800, or even in Galen's time, the hygienic prophylaxis and treatment of tuberculosis, its correlation with over-crowding and under-feeding, the importance of open air, good food and freedom from worry were as well known as in 1943. It is also true that the physicians of the eighteenth century were as well aware of the relation between putrid fever and slum conditions as we are. The new impulse came from the heart not from the head—the spirit of humanity, the rejection of the contemptuous fatalism which inspired the words of Galen I have quoted. Where, as I think, new intellectual knowledge contributed to the social betterment was by its educational value.

The theoretical schemata by which our ancestors 'explained' the diffusion of Typhus or the relation of Phthisis to over-crowding and under-feeding were hopelessly vague, they were academic in the bad sense of the word. To be able to demonstrate experimentally that tuberculosis was an infectious disease, to be able to show the *materies morbi* on a plate, living and multiplying; that gave people new hope and confidence. The enemy was not some vague abstraction, some ghostly miasma, but a tangible living foe to be fought and conquered. Common people were heartened to insist upon the carrying out of old and sound advice. They knew, or thought they knew, why that advice was good.

I am not seeking to insinuate that new scientific knowledge has not *directly* aided the prophylaxis and treatment of Pulmonary Tuberculosis; of course it has, everyone in the audience can think of examples. Then in acute infectious diseases, like Typhus, pure laboratory work has created an applied science of immunology which owes nearly everything to the experimental method. Those who exalt pure reason unduly may say that a first-rate reasoner might have deduced from centuries-old experience of smallpox inoculation, a complete science of immunology. Nobody did, however. Untested hypotheses, ingenious speculations, have no emotional drive. Experiments have. But even in the essentially modern triumph of active immunisation, there have been disappointments due to logical weakness whether in the interpretation of the data or, still more frequently, in the generalisation of correct inferences to groups not *in pari materia* with the experimental data.

Laboratory bacteriologists, field epidemiologists, even statistical epidemiologists, have often been led by their respective herd and individual vanities to claim special authority for their several methods of research. That is why epidemiology is still in its infancy; an imperfect co-operation of efforts each good. The authority of ancient books is dead, but the authority for which herd vanity and individual vanity hunger is alive.

I turn to the last of these Hydra heads of which I desire to speak—the authority of intention.

A few years ago, praise of scientific research for its own

sake would have been thought platitudinous in university circles and, if the speaker quoted the *Grammarian's Funeral*, banal. But recently men whose contributions to science pure and applied entitle their opinions on the organisation of science to respect have maintained that scientific research should be directed to the material and moral betterment of mankind, to the increase of man's control of his environment, and that the satisfaction of intellectual curiosity respecting problems which have no relevance to this social intention is, if not immoral, certainly no better than harmless amusement. They strongly advocate the planning of scientific research on lines guided by the authority of intention; in their view, Browning's *Grammarian* wasted his life. Those who dissent from this faith see danger to scientific freedom and *ad captandum* arguments are freely used by both parties.

To derive secret—sometimes even expressed—pleasure from the thought that one's investigations are remote from the interests of common men, and can only be judged by a select minority, is a less aggressive form of vanity than to decry those who do what we do not want to do, but it remains vanity and not a cardinal virtue.

The historical fact that a great majority of fundamental discoveries have been made by inquisitive men of genius who were just satisfying their curiosity is not a conclusive argument. Down to our own time, pleasing oneself was the only incentive to research in many branches of science; it would have been as difficult to persuade Mr Gladstone to spend public money on experimental entomology as to induce Sir Robert Walpole to endow chemistry. It is *not* true that a utilitarian impulse never stimulates the growth of pure science. Forty years ago, few young mathematicians were interested in biostatistics and none in industrial applications of statistical methods. A technological demand for biometricians and industrial statisticians has changed this. Some who supplied the demand have made fundamentally important contributions to the general theory of mathematical logic. Without invidiously selecting recent and living examples, one may cite Alexis Chuprov [8] who, in the opinion of better judges than I claim to be, ranks among the greatest exponents of the theory of statistical reasoning. But Chuprov was not a professional mathematician and took a practical interest in demographic and agricultural data. Planning science, in the sense of attracting or even compelling young men and women of ability to serve an apprenticeship in the human or humanly important applications of science, ought to increase technological efficiency and need not sterilise the creative impulses which produce the finest results of pure science.

But this argument goes no further than to show that, under planning, good work may be done. Authoritarian planning could only be the ideal system if we attribute to the planners a superhuman prescience, just as authoritarian political government is only an ideal system if the wielder of authority is all-wise. Let us accept the proposition that, if education had been planned on utilitarian lines a century ago, our material command of the environment would be greater than it is; it is still true that we should have lost much which, even from the purely technological point of view, has been of enormous value. Charles Darwin and Francis Galton as young men would not, perhaps, have found a patron. Mendel's interest in peas might have seemed frivolous. It is a commonplace of scientific history that discoveries made for the satisfaction of pure intellectual curiosity have often proved materially valuable to mankind. I will not cite examples familiar to the whole audience, but confine myself to one, not yet of outstanding importance, which has an association with Linacre.

The only work of Linacre (9) which has been reprinted within living memory is his translation of Galen's *de Temperamentis*. Galen probably valued this more highly than any other of his writings. Possibly because it is the shortest of his larger books, it is the least unknown of them; perhaps also because it discusses a problem which can never lose interest. A less intelligent physician than Galen would have perceived that human temperaments, psychological and corporeal, vary and that temperament is a factor of medical prophylaxis, diagnosis and treatment. Where Galen differed from his predecessors and successors (down to our own time) was in his insistence on the continuity of temperament, his refusal to admit absolute distinctions, and his desire to quantify the study. The traditional doctrine of opposite qualities—the hot and the cold, the moist and the dry—he used as a frame of reference. For him every human temperament could be represented by a point in a plane the position of which is determined by its co-ordinates (the origin is the ideal point, the perfect crasis). So the universe of human temperaments will be a frequency surface in the statistical sense. Galen did not, of course, express this geometrically but verbally and verbosely. His successors ignored his insistence on continuity and picked out 'typical' temperaments; hence one has the nine temperaments, viz. the perfect temperament, denoted in Galen's system by a point, the four simple excesses, denoted by points on the axes, viz. $(+x, 0)$ $(-x, 0)$ $(0, +y)$ $(0, -y)$ and the four linked excesses, viz. all the points in the four quadrants. Even this was too much, the nine temperaments dwindled into four, the choleric, sanguine, phlegmatic and melancholic, which survived the oblivion of the humours and qualities and still live. Galen's insistence on continuity was forgotten by clinicians.

Within the last century, pathologists have studied bodily temperaments and the Italian school of Giovanni, Viola and others tried to define bodily types in quantitative terms. Modern Italian statisticians, notably Marcello Boldrini[10], have sought to relate anthropometric indices of groups to indices of natality or mortality. The work of Jung and Kretschmer, not characterised by refined statistical technique, but showing great clinical insight, is famous. But it has been mainly to psychologists of the English and American schools that we owe a partial realisation of Galen's idea. The work arose out of primarily technological needs, the testing of intelligence. At first this was a relatively simple process, but it soon became clear that to characterise intelligence not one but many tests were needed. A brilliant suggestion of Spearman, his postulation of a general cognitive factor, enormously stimulated interest. These earlier researches were concerned with cognitive processes, but it was soon realised in measuring mind that the conative aspect of man's psyche could not be ignored.

So the wheel has come full circle; temperament is an object of quantitative study. Galen may look down from Elysium on the work of our investigators with a grim smile of approval. Possibly he may reflect that if *de Temperamentis* is hard reading (as it is), modern research papers employ a notation which all physicians do not find self-evident. Matrix algebra is not yet a compulsory subject for medical students; but text-book writers on factorial analysis prescribe a study of it for their readers (11). We no longer think that human temperament is defined by a point in a plane. We do not stay content with one or two measurements, we require a matrix of measurements and so must have recourse to the work of the mathematical logicians who studied matrices and their algebra because that study interested them.

It would have seemed strange indeed to Binet, Cauchy, Jacobi and Cayley had it been suggested to them that their investigations would have a technological interest for field psychologists immersed in the business of choosing careers for children or children for careers and might even come to have importance in the study of disease. Only a very prescient planner would have encouraged matrix algebra a century ago.

I do not wish to exaggerate the immediate practical importance of all this or to suggest that we are within sight of a satisfactory solution of the clinical and social problems which the variation of bodily and psychological temperaments presents. I do suggest that methods of investigation derived not from experimental but logical research now enable us to formulate the problems precisely; precise formulation of a problem is not a sufficient but a necessary condition of its solution. Technology, and medical research in the ordinary citizen's connotation of the term is technology, usually waits on 'pure' science, by which I mean the earnest pursuit of an intellectual curiosity, however remote from human interests that curiosity may seem to be.

I hope and believe that to a great majority of the audience the last sentences are truisms; that we all agree that medical research is intellectually more than technology. But certainly we might have expected that medical research workers would be less well defended against the authority of technologically minded planners than other investigators. Here surely the voices of sufferers demanding relief from pain or the postponement of death will be heard and will not encourage a parliamentary authority to spend money on 'academic' research.

There are two reasons why 'pure' research in medicine in our country is not much hampered by technological bias.

The first is that the science of medicine is, and has long been, ahead of its administrative practice. Scientific knowledge a generation old is still not applied, and cannot be applied because administration cannot be in advance of and usually lags behind the best informed public opinion of the day.

The other reason is that in the infancy of state-aided or endowed medical research in our country, administration was inspired and largely carried out by a public servant whose faith in intellectual freedom never faltered.

Walter Morley Fletcher's affection for Cambridge was passionate; emotionally he perhaps dichotomised mankind into Cambridge men and others; he may even have cherished a belief that Trinity was more blessed than other Colleges. But a man of any university or of none, with ideas, had as interested and encouraging a listener as one of Fletcher's foster brethren. The only men against whom he reacted with almost embarrassing violence were the Seeming Wise. 'Some, whatsoever is beyond their reach, will seem to despise or make light of it, as Impertinent or Curious; and so would have their Ignorance seem Judgment.' Such men, however important their station, found no mercy, in spite of the fact that Fletcher's social philosophy was hardly of the left wing. He fought for and secured a scientific freedom in state-aided medical research for which those who have enjoyed it bless his name.

It was said of the greater William Pitt that no officer left an interview with him without a conviction that my

Lord Chatham was the first man in the Empire and the interviewed the next greatest. There are many workers, perhaps some in the audience, who went disheartened to see Fletcher, feeling that their research was not going well, that they had over-rated their ideas. They left him heartened. His interest, his quick movements, even his characteristic stammer, gave one courage.

Thomas Linacre, possibly, Walter Fletcher, certainly, were in key positions, each at the beginning of a new epoch. It is not, I think, fantastic to see an analogy between their careers.

Perhaps Linacre did look backwards too wistfully, but there are, as I have tried to show, reasons for a charitable interpretation. It was said of Fletcher, by some clinicians, that he too looked backwards, that he unduly exalted the claims of the laboratory sciences in which the Cambridge of his youth and manhood had won spectacular triumphs and that he was intellectually contemptuous of clinical research. As a generalisation the charge is false, but Fletcher *was* impatient of rhetoric and did value measurements more than authoritative opinions. That was why he fostered the growth of the biostatistical techniques which, with all their limitations, do help to control the whimsical effects of herd and individual vanities; the authority of the Faculty or of the eminent individual. Fletcher did move slowly here, laying foundations on which to build clinical and sociological research, before seeking to organise such research.

In the Medical Research Council's series of Special

Reports are many concerned with the problems of what is now called Social Medicine; as examples I would cite No. 101, on Child Life Investigations, and No. 114 on Social Conditions and Acute Rheumatism; they illustrate —often by success in reaching, sometimes by failure to reach, a clear-cut conclusion—the virtues and defects of our methods. The doing of this unspectacular, careful work has prepared the ground for a future harvest. Clinical and sociological research had a better friend in Fletcher than most of its advocates realised.

Linacre is to us hardly more than a name; Fletcher a vividly personal memory. But, unless his story is told, Fletcher will become as shadowy as Linacre; administrators are soon forgotten. I, who gratefully remember many acts of generous kindness, cannot repay them by doing him full justice; my knowledge is not complete. I like, however, to think that to couple his name with that of Linacre in a Linacre Lecture, would have pleased him; a lecture in Cambridge which commemorates an Oxford scholar may fitly end with a tribute to a son of Cambridge.

REFERENCES

(1) J. N. Johnson, *The Life of Thomas Linacre*, London, 1835, p. 310.

(2) Unless otherwise stated, references are to the edition of Galen's work (text and Latin translation), edited by D. C. G. Kühn, printed at Leipzig, 1821–33. The only complete work of Galen translated into modern English, *On the Natural Faculties*, appeared in the Loeb Series in 1916. The translator, Dr A. J. Brock, in his *Greek Medicine*, London (Dent), 1929, has included some extracts from other works which throw light on Galen's characteristics.

(3) M. Greenwood, 'Galen as an Epidemiologist', *Proc. Roy. Soc. Med.* 1921, XIV (Sec. Hist. of Med. 3–16).

(4) M. Greenwood and M. Smith, 'Some Pioneers of Medical Psychology', *Brit. Journ. of Med. Psychology*, 1934, XIV, pp. 1–30, 158–91.

(5) Galeni *de Placitis Hippocrates et Platonis*.... Recen. et explan. G. Mueller, vol. I, Lipsiae, 1874.

(6) M. Greenwood, A. B. Hill, W. W. C. Topley and J. Wilson, *Experimental Epidemiology*. M.R.C. Special Report Series, No. 209, London, 1936.

(7) Wade Hampton Frost, *Papers* edited by K. F. Maxcey, New York, 1941.

(8) L. v. Bortkiewicz and others, 'Biographical Notices of A. A. Chuprov', *Nordisk Statistik Tidskrift*, 1926, V, pp. 161–96.

(9) *Galeni Pergamensis de Temperamentis, et de inaequali intemperie Libri Tres Thoma Linacro Anglo interprete....* Impressum apud praeclaram Cantabrigiam per Ioannem Siberch. Anno. M.D. XXI.

This was one of the earliest books printed at Cambridge. It was re-issued in facsimile, with an introduction by J. F. Payne, in 1881.

(10) M. Boldrini, *La Fertilità dei Biotipi*, Milan, 1931.

(11) G. H. Thomson, *The Factorial Analysis of Human Ability*, London, 1939. C. Burt, *The Factors of the Mind*, London, 1940.

Lightning Source UK Ltd.
Milton Keynes UK
UKHW010616081019
351208UK00001B/7/P